Soap Making

Organic And Natural Soap Recipes

Table of Contents

Introduction

Creating your personal soap is of fun. I love making my personal soap for myself and also giving it as presents to friends and family. Here's a short description of the three different soap making processes if you're thinking about making your soap however not sure the place to start:

1. Cold Process

Cool process soap making is making soap from scratch. The three simple elements you'll need to create soap by doing this are water, oils and sodium hydroxide (lye). Lye is classified as being a hazardous material. It might burn skin on contact.

When working with lye, you should be extremely thorough and take all safety precautions, for example wearing protective gloves, safety glasses, clothing, and shoes. Also, you must make sure you utilize a stainless saucepan and also have individual pots for soap making, etc. simply for your saving of lye and measure cups.

It is extremely important you employ an excellent recipe if making soap in this manner that lets you know most of the precautions you must consider when using lye; such as combining the water and lye outside or in an exceedingly well-ventilated area. The mixing of water and lye first produces a vapor so dangerous that it could burn your lungs.

When handling lye, you need to be very responsible plus it does sound intimidating, so a great deal of soap making beginners prefer beginning making their soap by the following two approaches.

2. Hand milled Method

This technique involves the grating of readymade soap (so there's no lye to bother about) that's subsequently melted with extra water. You could add your personal chemicals, for example, flower petals, herbs, lavender, oatmeal, spices, soap colors, and fragrance. Then you serve it into soap shapes and keep to create. To two weeks it will take up for a truly hardened soap although this may take twenty-four hours.

3. Burn and Fill Process

In my experience, here is the easiest way to utilize if you should be a novice. Burn and put soap comes in readymade soap blocks (no lye to deal with). It merely melts, sometimes inside the stove or double boiler, add your soap color, perfume and recommended chemicals, fill it into the form and leave it to set for a few hours. Once it's set it's willing to use!

While making soap by any of the techniques above, it is important, so you have the measurements of the soap, colorings, scents and chemicals right you use a superb formula. Additionally, it is essential when dealing with a hot, melted soap mixture that you do not accidentally splash on yourself.

Soap making is addictive. You do not wish to stop as soon as you make your first successful group! So why not get started on your soap making voyage today?

Chapter 1 – Learning how to make soap

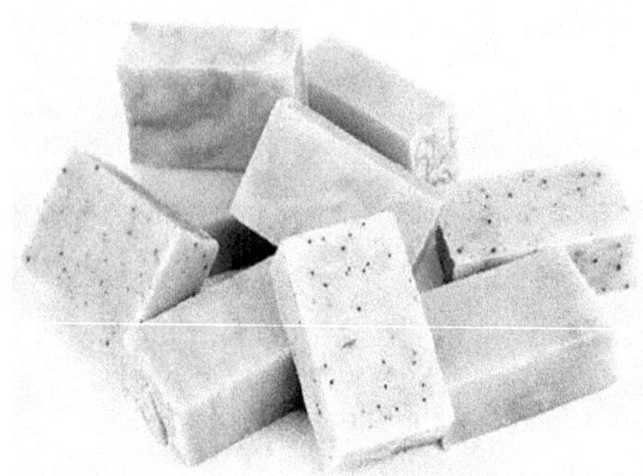

Learn to create a pure soap with minimal training. Adding lye and combining it with oils isn't that hard. After all, that's all that soap is real, it's a combination of oils and lye.

The procedure gets complicated by many attempts to explain it in confusing aspect with often conflicting ideas.

Listed here are a couple of tips to make sure to log off to a great begin with soap making.

It does not take plenty of peculiar pieces to create a soap that is wonderful. Look for recipes to get started which contain just a few simple components. It is difficult to a mix that is best that just involves olive and palm oils, grape, along with lye and water's right amounts too.

What is more, wholesale soap supply sites ensure it is easy to get your hands on these. With just those easy components, you can build soap that looks and feels like the most magnificent of soaps and all for not a lot of trouble or money either for example.

No components are required to create fabulous soap products.

If the basics don't work then, anything is much more work must be achieved by the method of making soap or even the formula is flawed and terribly wrong.

One key aspect in soap dishes may be the proportion of lye. It is included in the phrase lye discount.

Basically, which means that will be required to switch all your oils to soap applying less lye. And you likely don't wish to switch all of the oils to soap. You probably need a small bit of fat still unreacted to impart that luxury experience.

Having the lye amount right is easy once you know how to accomplish nevertheless it should be too low or not excessive and perfect both. Then there is the smell issue.

Many soap dishes, when made into soap, is going to be unscented while you set precisely what was needed while in the formula you've. You still get no scent or little and devote the total amount specified in the formula. A pity, since which means you still got nothing to exhibit for this but wasted the price of the odor.

For essential oils in freezing process soap, you may need about 0.7 ounces of acrylic per pound of soap. Which will be much more and less for mint and spice oils. And most citrus oils will not work nicely anyway. You can try acid oil fragrance, but just a few will experience the soap making process.

Use oil that is too much aroma, and it surely will remain free inside the soap. Too little won't smell whatsoever.

It's quite simple to learn how to make normal soap from soap making trial, and textbooks and error. The basics are very easy. Going beyond the basics, to experience quality massage soap, or to build soap to promote through a soap business, implies expertise and more study.

1.1   Problems which occur while soap making

I would prefer to tell you while making homemade cosmetics and especially soap, about one of the most prevalent problems that may arise. The approach of the making of handmade soap demands knowledge and reliability of some peculiarities of factors used. Nonetheless, although some of the guidelines might not be easy to comprehend without the exercise, you should know them.

So let's begin with the easiest mistakes which may arise during development of handmade soap in the soap base plus they are the next:

1.Accident avoidance throughout the work with the soap base. It appears to become absurd but it is not frivolous since highly heated foundation can cause burns, especially when it had been heated in the microwave oven.

2. While using the oils and flavoring agents, you ought to be careful. It's not recommended to mix these elements in a pan that are meant for food. Otherwise, soap-maker may encounter serious problems with medical. The factor is that flavoring agents could contain chemicals which kidneys and affect the liver. Essential oils may cause severe allergy. Consequently, so that you can be secure, you should find out the information about the ingredients you're likely to include.

3. Before starting the process of soap making, you have to know for sure what effect you're expecting. The newcomers should accompany this concept. Since in the beginning you'll need to work fast it is more straightforward to make a note of the sequence of activities. For example, English soap base solidifies quickly and due to the lack of experience you may be confused. It could lead to the truth that you can add the incorrect element.

4. Soap platform shouldn't be boiled or overheated. Factory soap base becomes dull under high-temperature and loses water. Consequently, we obtain soap of poor quality. So that you can prevent evaporation of water it is easier to warm the base on a water bath. It allows regulating the process better.

5. The concept of temperance. Often first soap makers generously put in a lot of colorants and essences to their soap. Such efforts of making their soap fresh and wonderful can lead to frustration.

It all arises from the lack of temperance. The too-large sum of colorants inside the soap can color the skin which can not be somewhat pleasant. Also, saturated colors in several split soap may slowly color the simple levels. Extra oils and vitamins that are not useless will appear as falls in the soap base. The issue is that the bottom doesn't recognize a lot of fat.

6. You do not have to include water into the soap base. It's not going to be valuable since water will only slow down the process of solidification of the soap. In the event if you'd like to produce your soap more beneficial and healthy you can fit a paper-bag with herbs to the foundation as well as in ten minutes it will be brewed just as within the water.

Attributes of some chemicals for the soap

The soap is melting perfectly.

Cinnamon and vanilla powder won't provide the scent that you will be wanting. Vanilla can only just offer a yellow tone towards the soap.

Therefore, it is better to enhance with soap flowers, you can surprise having a natural color.

Hibiscus blooms are also not useful except getting gray on their own since they do not give any shade.

Salt-added into the homemade soap has some peculiarities too. It quickly solidifies the soap base, and its particular crystals will appear on the soap's surface. Furthermore, food colorants ca n't color soap that was salty.

Excellent green doesn't provide fill natural color.

Caffeine powder or dried herbs can become as a harsh wisp. The coffee liquid does not supply the coffee odor.

Of course, this listing of basic mistakes isn't whole, and some more goods may be added, but develop that having learned these versions you'll avoid any disappointments, and the process of soap making will be nice and straightforward for you.

Chapter 2 – Process of Soap Making

For securely making custom made soap it is fundamental that the particular extents of these soap fixings are conscientiously taken after.

It is exceptionally suggested that you utilize a specific programming to figure the extents for every fixing and to run it each time another recipe is attempted. There are numerous sorts of virtual products for this reason. There are even iPhones applications.

Some fundamental gear must be utilized when planning soap fixings and making soap:

- a precise scale;

- a precise speedy perusing thermometer;

- a couple of little measuring cups; a stick blender to mix the oils with the lye blend and begin the saponification process;

- And soap molds.

Here is a case of the extents for the different soap fixings:

- 450 grams of vegetable fat;

- 170 milliliters of water

- 60 grams of burning pop

The soap making process

Arrangement of soap fixings

Soap making requires water, burning salt and fats or oils.

It is critical that burning pop is delicately poured into water, and NEVER the inverse which will bring about a sort of blast and sprinkle destructive item on your body. The temperature of the water and pop blend normally ascends to around 190°F or 90°C.

In this manner, a glass (Pyrex) or a stainless steel compartment is to be utilized. Try not to utilize a plastic holder as it would melt because of high temperature. It will be ideal if you recall that pop erodes aluminum. Continuously utilize wooden spoons to blend pop.

Blending the soap fixings

The pop temperature must let down to 95-105°F (35-40°C), and oil must be warmed up to 130°F (55°C). After checking those temperatures with a precise brisk perusing thermometer, gradually pour burning pop into the warmed oil. When the two fixings are blended, you can utilize a stick blender to mix the oil with the lye blend. While mixing the lye-water-oil blend with the stick blender, you turn on the blender in short blasts. Mix for 3 to 5 seconds and then mix some more.

When you begin utilizing the stick blender, you may see the oil turn shady, and the soap blend starts to meet up. Continue mixing in short blasts until the oil and lye water are totally combined. This ought not to take more than 30-40 seconds.

Presently you are nearing the stage called "follow." Utilizing the stick blender empowers you to achieve follow in less than a moment while If you utilize a wooden or a plastic spoon, it will take 10 to 75 minutes for the same result.

2.1 Hot Process Method for soap making

You'll find two major ways to produce soap and these are the soap making freezing process and hot process. The warm process of making soap has been an old practice in soap making.

Use heat and all that's expected within this approach is to set all the elements needed for soap making together in a pot. The important difference between this process and also the cool process may be the continual application of heat to make the soap. This technique of cooking produces harder soap bar than cold process method and quickens the process of soap configuration.

Whenever you start the soap making method that is hot, you'll not need so long on your side to begin any impromptu planning. You must, therefore, be ready with methods and all substances you will require. You should have all your security facilities like your hand-gloves, your ground your facemask and table includes ready. Crockpot, water, spoon, form, considering scale, blade, and other gear should be available.

The components ought to be assessed out based on the formula you have chosen. You may want to produce do with only a few additives to begin with. When you improve your soap making ability, it is possible to choose to include other elements.

Placed on gloves your facemask and glasses. You can also put on an extended sleeve clothing to safeguard your hand. You can now assess the Lye put it carefully into water mixing it at the same time. You have to blend until the Lye is totally mixed in the water. Always remember that Lye is what should be added to not one other way round and water.

Pour into the crock pot and permit it to dissolve. Now carefully fill the lye solution to the box of oils and continue to blend. This involves a steady stirring of the mixture. The combination while you proceed to stir may convert creamy then opaque. Keep stirring until trace or the mix begins to thicken.

The time the soap gets to this point put the lid on the pot and leave to make for a time. The soap will start to switch gel look that is clear like Vaseline. When the soap becomes to the look, it is time to test to confirm when it is prepared.

Now you can incorporate the soap mixture and perfume and the color of choice. After this, you could add your choice essential oils. You may need to do easily every one of these so that the soap combination does not cool to the stage it becomes quite difficult to get into the mold out of the box.

As it will soon be solid like custard, you will need to deal the blend out of the pan. Touch the form to make sure that any contained air is introduced. Allow the soap lower and to cool it after removing it in the mold into sizes and desired shapes. Virtually every instant focus is required by the process since the mix may remain in the container throughout the process. It is also extremely hard to make use of this technique as it is dangerous and fine to show children. However, unlike making soap's cool process, the soap making hot process delivers soap in a used format.

2.2 Cold Process Method for soap making

Soap can be used every day, making this skin care solution a simple product in supermarkets. Over the overall knowledge in the numerous brands soap, the components employed and the strengths of deploying it, what process is involved in making soap? One of the many soap making techniques is called cold process.

In soap making, freezing process is a fast and easy approach. When you are property, in reality, it may be completed. What makes cool process soap making popular with soap producers is its ease that it simply takes a little preparation. It's an operation that is best for generating health soap bars. Those who made it happen before may declare this of making soap as a favorite approach. While achieving this strategy, you may also integrate your imagination.

There are several freezing process measures. See the guidelines first. Work in a position that is properly ventilated and roomy. It is far better to possess a nearby stove and an ample water supply. Prepare using the warmth region to great and heal the soap when the products are total. Subsequently, put up and additives. Measure color and the extract if you would like and prepare decorative pieces.

Place and prepared the shapes oils and cosmetic specks within the stove. This can be done to make specks attachment and soap base and decrease temperature difference that occurs while investing in extra substances for the soap base.

The soap base components are being gauged by third means of freezing process without error. Inappropriate dimension can result in acid soap. Plus, incorrect quantity cause offensive soap tracing and may result in lye content and more gas.

In the oven, the temperature the lye compound as well as the oil. Last, cold process soap making process can require combining those two essential ingredients together.

You have to stir the resulting mixture from time to time. Fifth, devote the additives and then serve the soap mixture within the molds. Blend the materials immediately to avoid severe thickening. Setaside for a day to produce the soap molds arrives at a space temperature.

Cool process soap making also requires recovering. But before that, slice the homemade soap. Avoid as it can affect the soap in reducing any error. You're able to keep the soap intact in a dry and cool area, after which. Curing stays to get a minimum of a month and maximum of six.

Chapter 3 – Skin problem solutions with soap making

You may make soap to aid with many sorts of skin problems. The purpose for that skin is really because there's not that making soap is definitely better aren't harsh ingredients and the extra compounds. Regardless of what sort of soap, bought from handmade or the shop, are just a few components, fat, water or other liquid like goat's milk and lye.

You should use a several sorts of coconut oil essential oils, and avocado oil. With the addition of seed oil you may also protect your soap normally.

Because of this variance of components to generate soaps, a huge range is of soaps to assist with skin irritations. There would be a good idea to include chocolate butter for the combination, this will help skin. You need to use tea tree oil to help with stretch marks, scars and skin rashes. Different sebum like olive oil will help with allergies, eczema and a variety of different issues. By putting ingredients like goat's milk for your soaps, these also, plus a lot more can be gently cared for.

You may make your personal soaps out of essential oils also, from herbs including basil, mint and Lavender, to nuts like nuts macadamia and many more. These all have already been known to help protect, recover and moisturize your skin.

You can find different what can be put into become insect repellant and a natural sun protection. Citronella is simply one of these of a natural fat which can be employed for rejecting an assortment of stinging and stinging insects. There's no worry about perfumes, dyes or harsh chemicals within your soap because all of these are totally natural, most of the aromas are from natural materials.

The internet is a superb tool for folks who make soaps. You'll find literally hundreds of different sites on the subject of handmade soap making, to recommendations on what sorts of ingredients to incorporate for unique healing properties or aromatherapy, from basic measures in the act.

There's a great deal of different information to the rewards of making and applying normal and homemade soap products. You're able to learn to create strong bars of soap together with liquid soap products.

In addition to having the ability to produce soaps for your own needs, with hand-made soap items are created by you with things that benefit others. Knowing people who have skin or other health issues, you possibly can make soap to assist them with one of these conditions. You may also create other spots, or soap to sell, whether in specialty stores, at craft shows. You can be truly innovative and put in place your personal website to sell your soaps from.

You can start to make your own soap. It's not difficult to find out how, entertaining to complete and can even be a little addictive, when you get started and begin to understand all the stuff you are able to do with handmade soap. Guess what happens all the components are and many of these are incredibly affordable, so you save yourself a truck weight of money every year not having to buy from merchants.

Chapter 4 – Recipes of Organic And Natural Hand Made Soaps

Here are a few recipes you might want to use while making Natural Hand Made Soaps:

Beginner Cold Process Soap Recipe

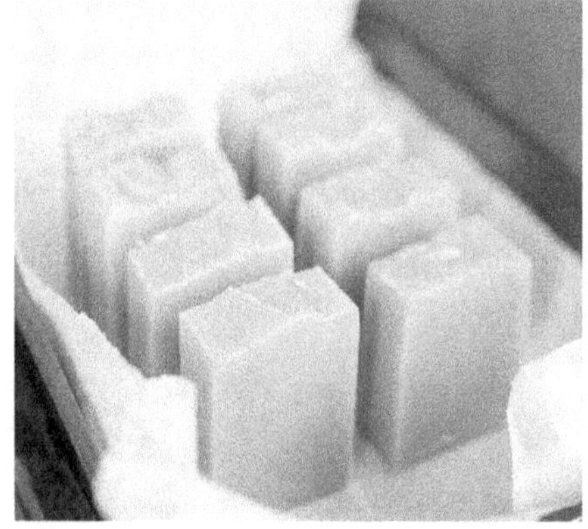

Ingredients:

15. palm oil

4 oz. coconut oil (76° melt level)

1 oz. castor oil

. fluid oz. Water

2.6 oz. lye/sodium hydroxide

1 – 1.25 oz. Optional, fragrance oil

Instructions:

By gathering all of your soap making equipment together begin. As well as your soap shape you'll also need a metal pan – no aluminum! – an electronic scale a stick blender, and different containers and utensils.

You'll then must follow than I'll below my fundamental cold process soap making training which moves a little more in depth and demonstrates photos of the steps. And don't use gloves and glasses as you're working together with lye and forget to consider proper safety precautions.

By calculating out the distilled water in fluid ounces begin. (I really used coconut water in my menu it did accelerate trace. You will need to chill it if you elect to mix the menu up a little and use water. It's also very important to note that it turns bright red if you incorporate the lye.) Pour into a pitcher.

Next, utilize a digital level to weigh out your lye. Make sure to have on all of your safety gear for this. Lye gets hot, and chemical burns will never be any fun. (in the event you get lye on your skin flush thoroughly with water.) Location the container you're using to assess the lye onto your size, push tare to zero it out slowly until you achieve the amount required, fill the lye into your package.

Slowly fill the lye in to the water, never one other way around as it could result in a not-so nice volcano effect. Mix your lye to the water with a wooden or plastic spoon until it melts. Now set away to cool. (If you're mixing the lye inside, maintain it about the range together with the fan turned on and step away. Or let it cool external to avoid the smells.)

Whilst the lye is chilling, burn and you'll need to weigh your oils. Mix the soap making oils into your metal box and heat to the oven over medium heat. (Alternatively you can even soften the oils individually in canning jars in a water bath.) Be sure while they may soften quickly to keep an eye about the fat. When they've melted take away the pot from temperature and invite to great.

Once the lye-water as well as the soap making oils have cooled to between 95°F-100°F you're ready to make soap.

Slowly put the lye-water in to the oils. Then, making use of your stay blender blend the lye- oils and water. You can add a fragrance oil if desired once your soap reaches a mild trace. Mix well to mix to some medium trace the serve the soap into your form that is ready.

Garden Mint Soap

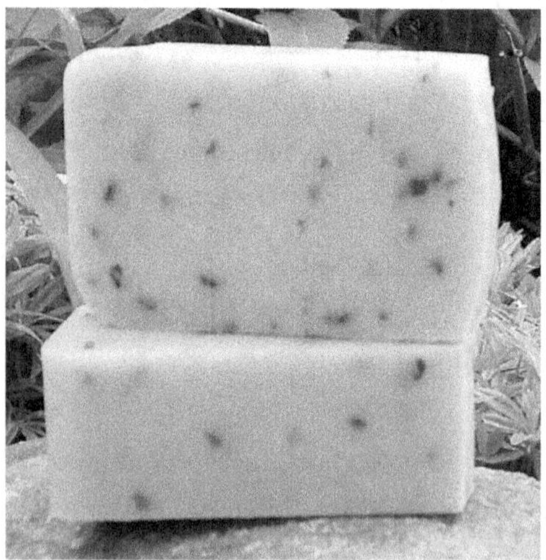

4 ounces Avocado Oil

24 ounces Coconut Oil

28 ounces Coconut Oil

4 ounces Castor Oil

2 ounces Mango Butter

9.0 ounces lye

19 ounces cooled mint-infused water (mint tea)

All dimensions are by weight. You must have a precise level to create soap.

To generate the water, add handfuls of clean (or dry) mint leaves to some vessel and serve simmering water over them. Transfer the bottle to the refrigerator, when it's cool enough to handle and invite it too high for a time longer.

At trace add:

1 1/2 tablespoons French green clay diluted with 3 tablespoons water

Two to three tablespoons (30 to 45 ml) peppermint essential oil

Pumpkin Soap Recipe

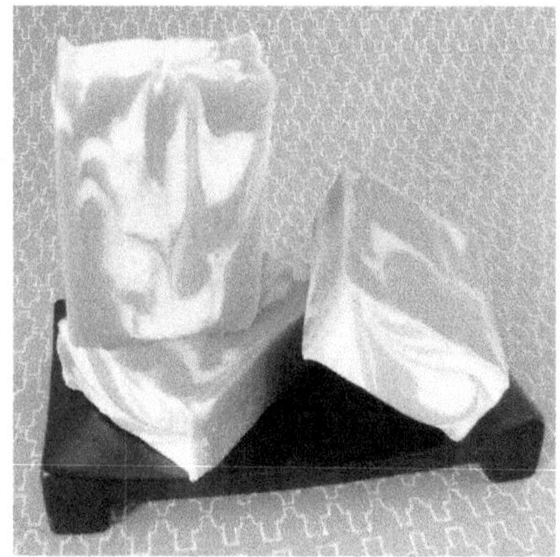

Liquid & Lye Percentage:

4.19 ounces lye

8 ounces distilled water

Oil Section (30 ounces total):

16 ounces' olive oil

8 ounces' coconut oil

3 ounces' sunflower oil

3 ounces' cocoa butter

At light track, merge:

2 ounces' pumpkin

Piece approximately 1/3 of the batter in a tiny plastic box out. Merge 1 tsp vanilla complete and 20 to 30 drops clove essential oil.

Fill half of the pumpkin soap to the parchment paper lined form, incorporate the vanilla spice layer then top using the rest of the pumpkin soap, next. Let and protect remain undisturbed for just two to three days.

Homemade Lemon Soap

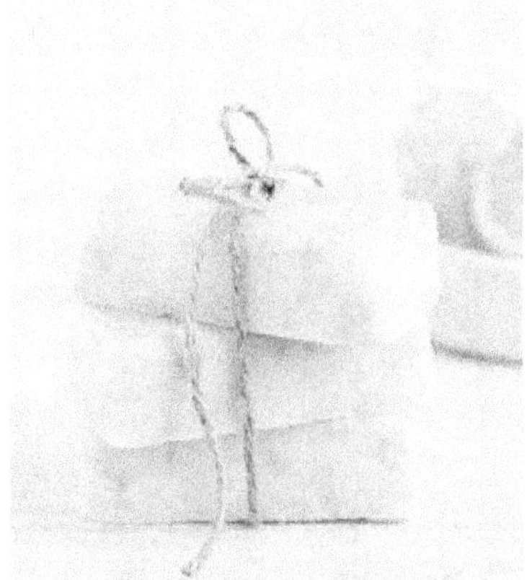

Ingredients:

1 1/2 cups Goats Milk cubed Soap Base

4-6 drops Lemon Gas

Dried Orange zest of 3-4 lemons

The 1st step: Reduce soap into cubes and microwave in 30 second periods (I love to employ a large Pyrex measuring glass to dissolve the soap in). This recipe makes 3-bars of soap and I used about 15 cubes of milk soap base that is goat's.

Second step: Dissolve soap for approximately one minute. If it's not completely melted, add another 15-30 seconds.

Step three: Once soap cubes have liquefied put in a few drops of the orange zest along with the orange essential oil; mix well.

Next step: Pour into soap molds and permit to harden for at least one time. Push mold to release soap.

LEMON BATH SOAP

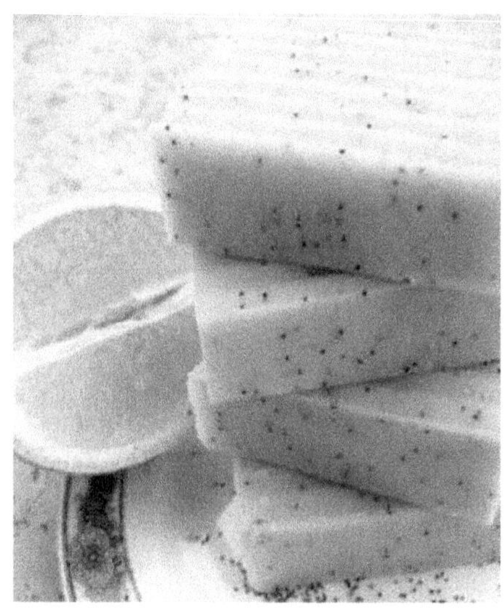

Ingredients:

1 cup baking soda

1/2 cup citric acid

1/2 corn starch

3 tablespoons epsom salt

3/4 teaspoon water

2 teaspoons Almond Oil

Lemon Gas

Yellow food dye (optional)

Wilton Icing Daisy

Plastic ornament mold

Meat Baller (optional)

The 1st step: In a big bowl combine baking soda, citric acid, cornstarch, and salt.

Step two: In a tiny bowl mix oil, water, color and oil.

Step three: put moist mixture into mixture. Blend using a stir until completely combined. Check mixture by pushing a handful together. Work with a spray container to SOFTLY spray water twice or once when the mix doesn't hold.

Avoid adding perhaps the blend or an excessive amount of water will fizz rather than form while in the mold correctly. Once it's the correct consistency click mixture into mold and permit before removing to dry at least 2 hours. Established a towel to dry with bath bombs.

LAVENDER CHAMOMILE TEA SOAP

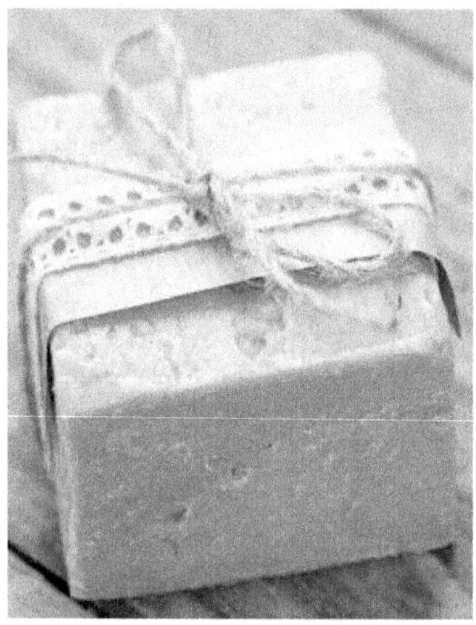

Ingredients:

Goats Milk Soap Base

Chamomile Tea (2 tea bags)

Lavender Gas

Lavender Flowers

Large Pyrex Pot

Silicone Mold

The first step: cut on 1 lb of the soap base into cubes. Location soap cubes in a big pyrex glass and dissolve over a boiler.

Second step: Mix in 10-15 drops of lavender gas to the melted soap. Stir in 1-2 tablespoons dried lavender flowers. This looks great mixed within the soap and will enhance the lavender smell. Immediately mix in dried chamomile tea leaves.

Step three: Pour into soap form and allow hardening for a few hours. Tip: should you see air bubbles on the surface you can apply them.

Rosemary Lavender Soap Recipe

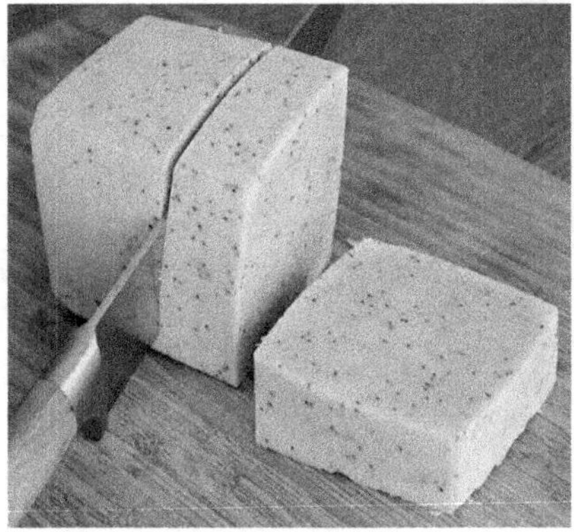

3 cups glycerin soap base

1/4 cup infusion of rose flowers and rosemary leaves

1 1/2 teaspoon, lavender oil

1/2 teaspoon rosemary oil

1 teaspoon pulverized dried rosemary

Herbal ingredients and mix melted platform, mix until mixed, then pour into great and shapes.

* Infusions are created by serving hot water over seed components, 3 tablespoons of dry or fresh plant per cup of water. Non- water is best.

Chapter 5 – Some more recipes

Organic Calendula Soap Recipe

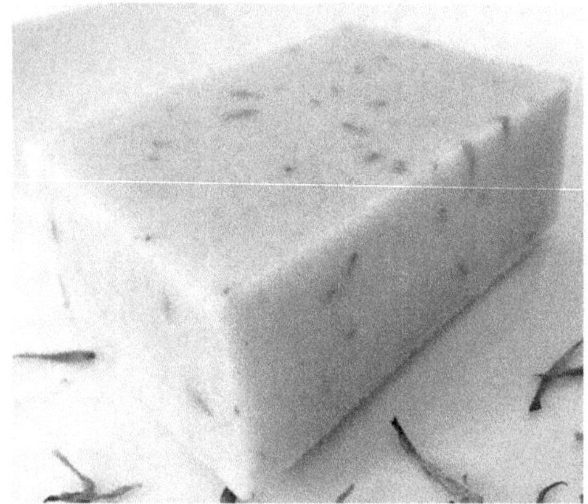

Makes a 454g/1 lb set – around. 4-5 bars.

120g (4.23oz*) boiling Water

64g (2.25oz) Sodium Hydroxide (Lye)

1 tsp (1g / 0.04oz) dried Calendula petals (2tsp if using fresh petals)

112g (3.9oz) Coconut oil

164g (5.78oz) Olive oil Pomace

82g (2.9oz) Tallow OR Palm Oil

78g (2.75oz) Sunflower oil

19g (0.67oz) Shea Butter

6 drops Grapefruit Seed Extract or Antioxidant – Large IU Vitamin E oil

*Please remember that all measurements are in bulk (consequently oz in beverages isn't fluid oz)

Method: Impress Calendula plants within the boiling water and invite before following basic soap making measures to cool to room temperature.

Herbal Soap Recipe

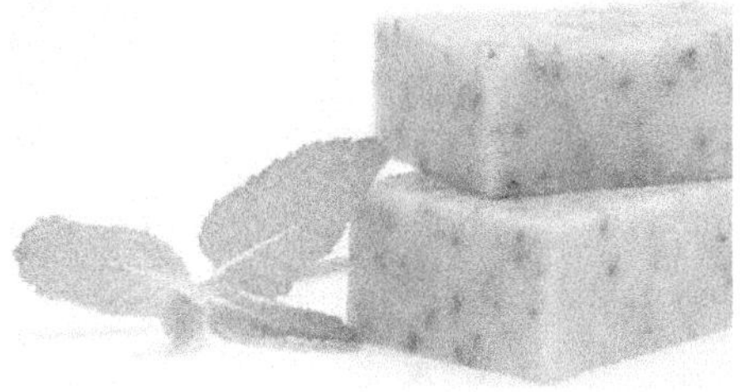

Makes a 454g/1 pound portion – around. 4-5 bars.

120g (4.23oz*) boiling Water

62g (2.19oz) Sodium Hydroxide (Lye)

136g (4.8oz) Coconut oil

204g (7.2oz) Olive oil Pomace

91g (3.2oz) Sunflower oil

23g (0.8oz) Shea Butter

10g (0.4oz) Essential oil (approx. 1 teaspoon) – Fit to your selected plant

Method: invite before following basic soap making actions to cool and Impress the herbs within the boiling water. Add gas at moderate track.

Natural Lavender Soap Recipe

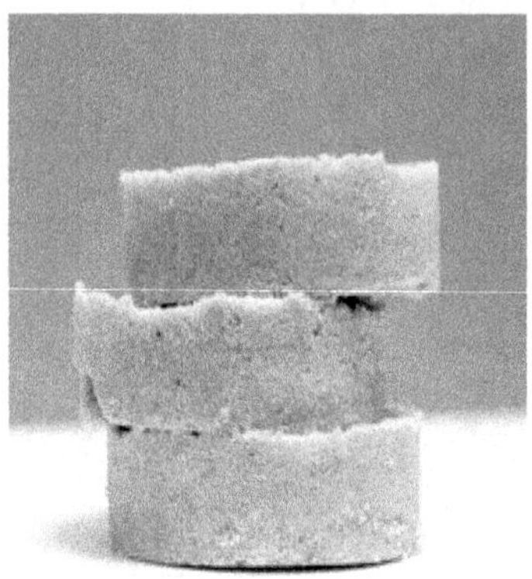

Makes a 454g/1 pound set

120g (4.23oz*) Water

64g (2.25oz) Sodium Hydroxide (Lye)

112g (3.9oz) Coconut oil

164g (5.78oz) coconut oil Pomace

82g (2.9oz) Palm Oil

78g (2.75oz) Sunflower oil

19g (0.67oz) Shea Butter

10g (0.4oz) Rose acrylic (approx. 1 tsp)

1/4 teaspoon (0.8g/ 0.003oz) Ultramarine Violet (optional spring shade)

6 drops Grapefruit Seed Extract or Antioxidant – High IU Vitamin E oil

*Please note that all dimensions come in mass (therefore oz in beverages isn't fluid ounce)

Process: Distribute the vitamin color within your oils with a tiny milk frothier before following basic soap making ways. Include gas and dry plants at moderate trace.

Baby & Oats Soap Recipe

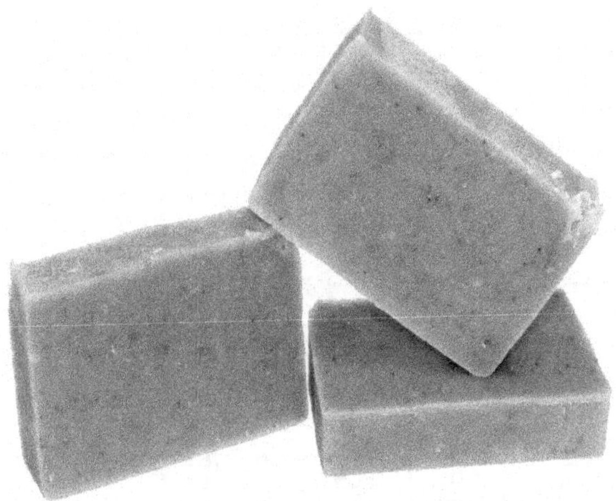

Makes a 454g/1 lb group – around. 4-5 bars. Super fatted

120g (4.23oz) Water

63g (2.22oz) Sodium Hydroxide (Lye)

136g (4.8 oz) Coconut oil

195g (6.9oz) Olive oil Pomace

68g (2.4oz) Castor oil

45g (1.6oz) Palm Oil OR Tallow

9g (0.32oz) Beeswax

1 tsp (2g / 0.07oz) Rolled Oats

Strategy: Add Honey in well at light track and whisk. Add oatmeal at moderate trace.

Choosing Your Oils

Soap will be the end product of an all-natural chemical reaction between oils (acids) and lye (a platform). You can't produce soap without either of these two kinds of components. The types and portions of oil you utilize within your soap will influence how much lye (Sodium Hydroxide) you'll require inside your menu

so let's focus on them.

Think about the most effective club of soap you've ever used. Achieved it has fluffy lather? Was it vulnerable? How difficult was the club? How did the skin feel afterward? The oils you choose inside your formula will have on what your closing soap will be like a massive impact.

Listed here are examples of sorts of oils which will donate to different aspects including hardness, washing, lather, and health. A terrific pub of soap may have an excellent balance of all of them, so it's recommend to select five and between three oils initially. The three oils to make a basic soap recipe is a combination of Palm Oil/Tallow, Olive Oil Pomace, and Coconut oil.

They're affordable and applied to their particular will generate a good bar that is balanced.

Using Palm oil in Soap making

A massive conflict in soap making companies around the use of Palm oil. Also known as plant-tallow, it has the same soap making properties as animal fat and is particularly very cheap.

Being also multipurpose, you'll find it used to biscuits towards the oil used to deep fry ingredients from Crisco, to chocolate, to everything. Should you see 'vegetable oil' or 'vegetable fat' and appear around the elements number of a food item it's very likely that the item contains Palm Oil.

Because of usefulness and its low-cost, Palm oil has now got to be the most used gas worldwide and it's now projected that 33% of all edible oil used is Hand. Due to the popular, offer has had to increase and

Rainforests across Australia are being cut and burned to produce more land to parking it. This has led to the damaging loss of habitat for pets including Orangutans, therefore, consumers and many suppliers now avoid it or items built using it.

Conclusion

Soaps are believed essential within our properties. It is unlikely that the particular property won't have any of these since these are virtually washing agents that people use.

These cleaning agents' use dates back to the historical times which have been maintained up to the current. Dramas are essentially useful for washing, cleaning and cleansing. These cleaning agents are synthesized from vegetable or pet fats. When it comes to washing, soaps are extremely efficient.

Soap making is mixing the garbage to be able to make the finished goods or just a matter. Of making soaps, the approach can also be known as saponification. This method essentially entails mixing fats and oils with a specific amount of alkali. In the formation of salts of essential fatty acids, this mix results in soap making.

These salts record the dust and oil making certain they will be removed from the surface. The dust and soap mix includes it, leaving just a clean area, as that is washed by water.

You can find various kinds of soaps that are made. Besides from your professional people that we are used to, additionally, there are handmade soaps. These handmade soaps will be the goods from making the soaps from scratch, that you get.

These two soaps' features are extremely different. In fact, making it entails super fatting or even the improvement of an extra quantity of fats to the soap mixture. The primary advantage of this technique would be to create the soap skin-friendly. It is still ready to maintain it moisturizing property since the glycerin is left untouched inside the soap.

There are various kinds of soap making processes. These would be warm process the cool process along with the put & burn process. There are particular advantages and disadvantages that these practices have.

The cold process is performed by slightly reducing the mixture preserve it at that temperature and to liquefy it. The hot method of soap making requires warming the soap mix into a higher temperature. For that melt & pour method, there is a pre-made mix which mixed and is melted into the shape.

Soap making is an easy approach for this is readily available because the fresh materials needed to accomplish. You will get them even and in your grocery stores in specialty hobby shops. Soap making is a flexible exercise to do. You're able to personalize the soaps that you simply produce determined by your taste. It's up to you to add the soaps' odor and also along with. Whatever it's you want, you possibly can make it with your soaps.

Imagination makes soap making extremely entertaining! You can do anything that you want with your soaps. Do not get too excited because there are certain precautionary measures that you should take whenever you make your soaps.

FREE Bonus Reminder

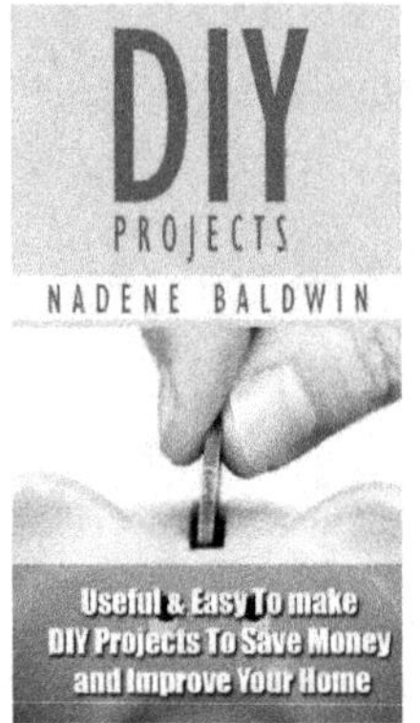

If you have not grabbed it yet, please go ahead and download your special bonus report *"DIY Projects. 13 Useful & Easy To Make DIY Projects To Save Money & Improve Your Home!"*

Simply Click the Button Below

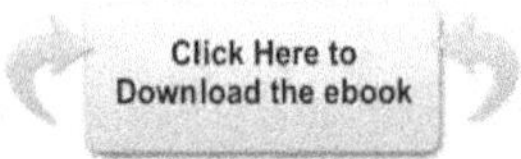

OR **Go to This Page**

http://diyhomecraft.com/free

BONUS #2: More Free & Discounted Books

Do you want to receive more Free & Discounted Books?

We have a mailing list where we send out our new Books when they go free or with a discount on Kindle. Click on the link below to sign up for Free & Discount Book Promotions.

=> Sign Up for Free & Discount Book Promotions <=

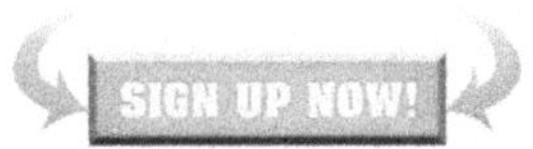

OR Go to this URL

http://zbit.ly/1WBb1Ek